Rural Clinician Airway Management (RCAM)

Rural Clinician Airway Management (RCAM)

A Practical Guide to Managing Airways in the Rural Setting

Samuel L. Marshall

ISBN-13: 9780692819722
ISBN-10: 069281972X
Library of Congress Control Number: 2017900347
Rural Clinician Airway Management, West Point,MISSISSIPPI

Disclosure

Every effort is made to provide current evidence-based medicine guidelines, and this lecture is intended for guidance only. This lecture material should never supersede clinical judgment, a state's scopes of practice, employing-agency policies, or medical standards of care as defined by your medical director. Your current instructor assumes no liability for clinical decision making or patient care provided by participants taking this course.

To my wife, Danielle—your love, patience, and encouragement gave me the motivation to continue this endeavor. I will never be able to thank you for the patience you have demonstrated in our marriage for my quirky ideas. Even though my grandfather (Erst) called you Diane, he was right when he said you were my best catch.

To my daughters, Maggie and Cate—you are my daily motivation to make a difference and remind me of the sweet faces I am attempting to protect.

To Mom and Dad, who believed in me even when I didn't. You never gave up on me—here's your result.

To Ben—your early departure inspired me to change the culture in airway management. You somehow still remind me to never forget the good times.

Contents

Acknowledgments

I OWE THANKS TO many different individuals for supporting me in this endeavor, and I know there are people I owe tremendous gratitude whom I might not mention. Dr. Lee Valentine and Angie Burkes of the EC-Healthnet Family Residency Program in Meridian, Mississippi, have been instrumental in supporting my cause of improving airway management. Without their support, this course and book would not have been possible, and for that I am grateful. Implementing my airway course in the EC-Healthnet curriculum has not only improved emergency training for the residence physician but also helped assist me with course improvements, making this available for other areas across the country.

My friends and coworkers in the emergency and air medical field have provided support and feedback that I am grateful to have.

Thanks go to Duke Johns of Medical Specialties in New Orleans for his continued support and wisdom. Duke gave me a new opportunity to see various viewpoints in health care and demonstrated that people who genuinely have the patients' best interests in mind do still exist.

Dr. Jason Farrar of the EC-Healthnet Family Residency Program in Meridian, Mississippi, was instrumental in validating the RCAM course by creating and implementing a study involving the resident physicians. I appreciate his passion and assistance helping improve this course.

This book was written with the intent to supplement a didactic lecture to improve critical thinking and airway skill management. The book is designed primarily using lists to complement associated lectures and enhance important aspects of the course. Although not every aspect of airway management is included, such as specific patient populations, the book is to enhance clinicians of all levels and influence the need for continuing education in this specific area. A self-study version is currently being designed and soon available for an individual learning experience.

Contributors

Cori L. Bitner, AGACNP-BC, CCRN, CEN, C-NPT
Flight Nurse
University of Mississippi Medical Center-AirCare
Jackson, MS

Patrick Barber, DO
EC-Healthnet Family Medicine Residency
Meridian, MS

Angela Bevill, DO
EC-Healthnet Family Medicine Residency
Meridian, MS

Moumita Biswas, DO
EC-Healthnet Family Medicine Residency
Meridian, MS

Matthew Capalbo, DO
EC-Healthnet Family Medicine Residency
Meridian, MS

Casey Copeland, RN, CEN, TCRN
Trauma Program Manager
Rush Foundation Hospital
Meridian, MS

Taylor Eisenmenger, DO
EC-Healthnet Family Medicine Residency
Meridian, MS

Jason Farrar, DO, MBA
EC-Healthnet Family Medicine Residency
Meridian, MS

Terry L Forrette, MHS, RRT, FAARC
Adjunct Associate Professor
LSU Health-New Orleans, LA

Jonathan Fuller, DO
EC-Healthnet Family Medicine Residency
Meridian, MS

Brad T. Harper, NREMT-P
Flight Paramedic
University of Mississippi Medical Center-AirCare
Jackson, MS

Hunter Harrison, DO
EC-Healthnet Family Medicine Residency
Meridian, MS

Gabriel Madu, DO
EC-Healthnet Family Medicine Residency
Meridian, MS

Casey N. Mancini, DNP, CRNA
Rush Foundation Hospital
Department of Anesthesia
Meridian, MS

Lindsey L. McCormick, DO
EC-Healthnet Family Medicine Residency
Meridian, MS

Chris Moore, DO
EC-Healthnet Family Medicine Residency
Meridian, MS

Samantha Mosby, DO
EC-Healthnet Family Medicine Residency
Meridian, MS

Jenisus Owens, DO
EC-Healthnet Family Medicine Residency
Meridian, MS

Matthew Roberts, DO
EC-Healthnet Family Medicine Residency
Meridian, MS

ShyAnn Shirley, RN, CEN
Flight Nurse
University of Mississippi Medical Center-AirCare
Jackson, MS

John Thames, DO
EC-Healthnet Family Medicine
Residency
Meridian, MS

Owen Ulmer, DO
EC-Healthnet Family Medicine
Residency
Meridian, MS

James L. Valentine, DO
EC-Healthnet Family Medicine
Residency
Director of Medical Education
Meridian, MS

Matthew Ward, DO
EC-Healthnet Family Medicine
Residency
Meridian, MS

Prologue

Airway management is a hot topic in emergency and critical-care medicine. You can go to almost any ambulance service, hospital, or local college and find airway and intubation mannequins for training and maintaining skill competencies. So why is airway management a common conversation in the emergency medical field but continues to be a poorly managed problem? Why is much emphasis placed on CPR training but not on the prevention of cardiac arrest? Much training in regard to airway management involves teaching a skill. The skill of intubation is learned by repetitive training, but without any critical thinking and team management involved. Paramedics graduating from school are generally competent in the skill of intubation, and they are often called to assist in other departments of a hospital, but any alteration of the intubation guidelines could cause havoc. Assessment of a potential difficult airway and changing the pharmacology choice are not generally taught to a new nurse, paramedic, or physician. After many conversations with instructors of medical schools, paramedic programs, and nursing schools, I have found that the primary focus is whether students pass the certification exam that is required for the school to maintain accreditation. The certification exams are generally how the instructor and school are graded on performance of instruction and accreditation. The old saying "The student knows just enough to kill someone" is a true statement in many cases. Schools have been forced to focus on graduating more exam-prepared students rather than students with critical thinking and skill. States do not require specific board certifications for physicians working in emergency departments, and most hospitals require the basic alphabet course, including Advanced Trauma Life Support. After much research, I have found there is little focus on airway training for staff working in the emergency department. This lack of training might explain why helicopters are frequently called for assistance.

This course is designed to prepare all clinicians working in the emergency department or prehospital environment for airway management. This course is not teaching a skill to students but rather assisting them in developing an ability to make conscious evaluations, implementations, and decisions to better manage patients and reduce sentinel events.

There are many organizations and societies focused on improving airway management that implement initiatives to help guide the practitioner. What seems to be lacking is the actual facilities employing clinicians providing attention on implementing any type of guidelines. A retrospective study focusing on rural critical-access hospitals noted that a vast majority of patients who required helicopter transport were intubated by the air medical personal, suggesting the use of air over ground transport. This study demonstrated that helicopters might be requested for a needed skill rather than a rapid transport to a tertiary facility.

Discussing standards of care related to airway management appears to be no different than other forms of medical treatment.

Although there are many guidelines published by reputable organizations, disclosures are clear identifying that the published guidelines do not constitute any standard of care, even though many perceive them in that manner. Unfortunately, this book is no different and only provides guidance to make informed decisions but does not replace or construe a standard of care.

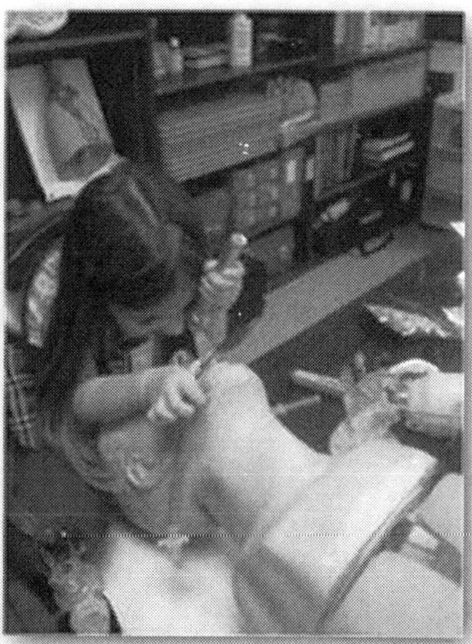

Figure 1 I taught my daughter the skill of intubation when she was six years old, and she almost mastered the skill even with underdeveloped muscles. I was unable to teach her critical thinking at a young age.

Bibliography

Henderson, K., L. H. Woodward, K. C. Isom, J. Wilson, and R. L. Summers. "Prevalence of Intubation Rescue by Air Medical Personnel during Transfers from Rural Emergency Departments." *Air Medical Journal* 34, no. 3 (2014): 141–43.

Hung, O., and M. F. Murphy. *Management of the Difficult and Failed Airway*. New York: McGraw-Hill Med, 2012.

1

Scenarios

THE SCENARIOS DISCUSSED below are to create an awareness of situations that can and do exist every day to help initiate the process of critical thinking. Every time a clinician is faced with an airway decision, the results can be polar opposites when comparing different mind-sets of the importance of being prepared for worst-case scenarios. When reading or discussing the below scenarios, picture yourself and current coworkers in this situation and think how you would react and manage.

Scenario One

You are called to the bedside of a six-year-old child admitted for acute chest syndrome secondary to a sickle-cell crisis. Upon arrival, you note the child sitting in a tripod position with increased work of breathing. Oxygen is currently being administered at 15 liters per minute via a nonrebreather mask. After receiving a report from the nurse and speaking with the child's mother, you make the decision to intubate due to the patient's hypoxia and hypercarbia.

You are concerned with impending respiratory failure and call for the rapid-response team for assistance. You perform what is (in your opinion) a common procedure and note the child becoming combative after administering medications. Medications administered are pretreatment fentanyl and induction agents midazolam and rocuronium. Your partner is unable to attempt intubation due to the child becoming combative. You note a sudden drop in oxygen saturation (SpO_2), and the child becomes lethargic with bradycardia.

Thoughts: Imagine yourself in this scenario.

- Was intubation appropriate based on the information given?
- What would be your next action?
- Do you have a systematic plan in place to mitigate adverse events like the scenario mentioned above?
- Why was there an immediate drop in oxygen saturation?

Scenario Two

You walk in the emergency department to start your night shift when you notice everyone in the trauma room. You receive a report that a thirty-seven-year-old male arrived by ambulance after being involved in an ATV accident. The patient is combative, and the physician is preparing to intubate. You note stable vital signs and the patient attempting to get off the hospital bed. The patient receives physician-ordered medications, and attempts to intubate the patient are made. The first intubation attempt is unsuccessful, and the patient's oxygen saturation starts declining. The staff prepares to ventilate the patient via bag-valve mask but is unable to find the face mask. The staff is unable to find a second mask, and the physician states the patient received a full dose of rocuronium. The obvious impending chaos is noted in the faces of the assisting staff frantically looking for equipment.

Thoughts:

- Was intubation appropriate with the information given?
- Imagine the panic in a small emergency department when the staff has this type of situation.
- Consider what options they had at that moment.
- Would having plans in place for alternative actions be helpful?

Every choice you make has an end result.

—Zig Ziglar

Scenario Three

You prepare to intubate a seventeen-year-old female who was thrown from a horse. The patient was brought to your local rural emergency department fully spinal immobilized by EMS. The patient presented with snoring respirations and a Glasgow Coma Score of 6. You order the routine medications of midazolam and rocuronium for intubation, and the patient begins to vomit when you attempt to advance the laryngoscope. The staff advises they are unable to get the suction unit to function, and it is hard to maintain a good seal with the BVM mask due to the amount of fluid around the mouth.

Thoughts:

- Was intubation appropriate with the information given?
- Was the medication choice appropriate for this patient?
- How would you handle a malfunctioning suction unit?

The goal of this book is to encourage clinicians and organizations to take responsibility and change the culture for better airway management by understanding the need for better education and equipment. Once the understanding is gained, implementation of an airway protocol with proper guides and equipment will result in better outcomes for the staff and patients. After reading this book or taking the course associated with this book, think about how you would handle the above scenarios differently. Having successful airway outcomes all starts with the proper education and preparedness, and having successful outcomes requires out-of-the-box thinking.

2

Early Considerations

WHY PREPARE? "I'VE already been to school" or "It is not my responsibility!" Most clinicians have heard or said something similar at some point in their careers. With financial reimbursement at an all-time low and the cost to provide medical care increasing, one can understand why many can't afford to take the time off for a conference or medical course, and hospitals do not have the educational budget to pay for such education. With the availability of Internet webinars and online educational offerings, the need for actual travel is far less than it was a decade ago, offering the clinician valuable resources. Regardless of your experience level, the lack of standardized airway equipment must be considered and evaluated when working at a new hospital or EMS service. Below are points to consider to better help you prepare and quickly analyze your department limitations.

Points to Consider for the New Nurse or Resident Physician

- No emergency department is standardized with the same staff or equipment.
- Consider time and distance to tertiary centers when needing to transfer a patient.
- Do you have surgery available? Are surgery staff members on call?
- Consider radiology availability. Do you have CAT scan (CT) and ultrasound?
- What airway equipment is available? Video laryngoscope? Ventilator?
- Are secondary or backup airways available?
- Are surgical airway kits available? Wired or scalpel?
- What airway medications are available? Are they located in the emergency department?
- Is respiratory therapy available?
- Identify the emergency department champion to be your assistant.
- Does the facility have a protocol or airway reference tool?

Be Prepared

There are many websites and books available for reference. Podcasts like Emcrit.org, by Scott Weingart, and Prehospitalmed.com, by Dr. Minh Le Cong, offer great updated research and blogs to help you improve knowledge and skill. Listening to a podcast is easy and certainly helps pass the time on a long road trip. Educational resources like the Society for Airway Management and Difficult

Airway Society provide helpful template guides and specific topics to be edited to fit the needs of your facility or service. Below are examples of free downloadable material to improve the preparedness for any clinician or facility.

Sample Checklist and Guide from SaferAirway.org

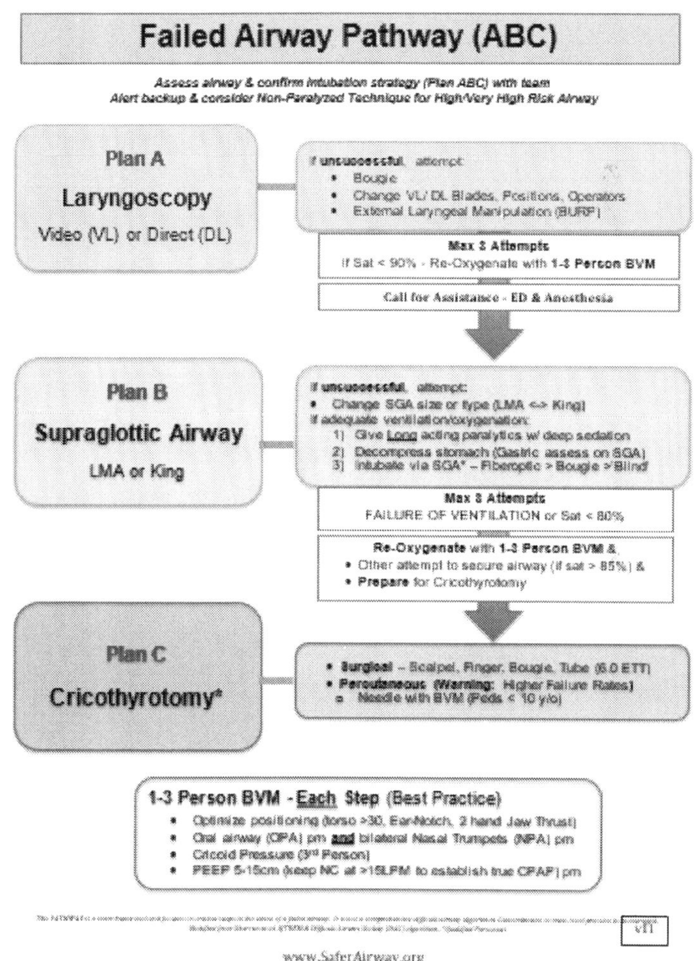

Safer Airway Checklist

Preperation Before Intubation ⇨ **During Intubstion** ⇨ **Post Intubation Protection**

Airway Assessment & Plan Shared?
(By Physician)
- ☐ Level of Difficulty (Specified Concerns)
  (Circle) Low, Moderate, High, Very High
- ☐ Plan ABC & Medications Needed
  - Plan A - "Primary" - DL/VL, Bougie
  - Plan B - "Backup" SGA (LMA/King) Size
  - Plan C - "Cricothyrotomy" Approach

Patient Ready?
- ☐ Monitor (Pulse ox, Card, BP, EtCO2)
- ☐ Positioning ("Ear to Sternal Notch")
  - ☐ "RAMP" if Obese
- ☐ Dual PreOxygenation (Both)
  - ☐ Nasal Cannula @ 15+LPM AND
  - ☐ NRB/BVM @ Flush

Equipment Ready?
- ☐ Bag & Mask on O2 & Suction Set Up
- ☐ Airway Cart & Glidescope Set Up
- ☐ ETT/syringe, SGA, & ____ on bedside Table

Medication Ready?
- ☐ Premedication (Prn)________
- ☐ Sedation/Induction________
- ☐ Paralysis (Prn)________

Intubation
- ☐ Time Out – Medication Nurse Assures "Everyone Ready"
- ☐ Announce "Beginning Intubation" (Give RSI Medication)
- ☐ Maintain Nasal Cannula at 15+ LPM
- ☐ Confirm Tube Placement
  - Auscultation
  - EtCO2 (Waveform preferred)

Post-Intubation
- ☐ Elevated Head of Bed 30-45°
- ☐ Continuous Waveform Capnography
- ☐ ABG in 10-15 min
- ☐ OG Tube Placement
- ☐ CXR
- ☐ Restraints per Intubation Protocol
- ☐ Sedation Orders
- ☐ **Debrief**
  1) "What went well?" ________ ☐See Back
  2) "What could be strengthened & how?" ________ ☐See Back
- ☐ **Difficulty Rating** (Post Intubation)

(Circle) Low, Moderate, *High, *Very High

For "High/Very High" Difficulty Ratings
- ☐ Bracelet on Patient
- ☐ Update Chart Problem List
- ☐ Communicate on sign out/transfer
- ☐ Airway Alert Letter completed by physician & in the Checklist Folder
- What made the Airway "Difficult"? ________ ☐See Back

Patient ID *(Sticker)*
Patient Name ....
ID # ....
Date .... Unit/Room ....

Team
Physician: ....
Nurse Lead: ....
Resp. Therapist: ....
Scribe: ....

QA
Attempt # (Circle) 1 2 3 4 5 +5
Precipitous/"Crash" Airway: ☐No ☐Yes
Any O2 Saturation < 90% ☐No ☐Yes
Device Used: ☐N/A ☐LMA ☐King ☐Cric ☐Flex Fib. Scope
Comments .... ☐See Back

Hospital Logo Here

This form is a QA tool and is **NOT Part of the medical record**. This checklist template is not intended to be comprehensive; customization to meet local practice and standards is encouraged.

www.SaferAirway.org

V 2017.2

Improving Airway Management: Team Approach

Improving airway management is a team effort and requires each team member to know his or her role when someone requires intubation. When dealing with certain scenarios such as pediatric patients, allowing the physician to be the only clinician making decisions can lead to failure and not using knowledge and experience of each clinician in the room.

Mental Toughness

Controlling the clinician's personal sympathetic response when dealing with airways can improve successful intubations. Many well-known airway experts discuss how early preparation for airway management reduces anxiety and fear. Having a checklist and guide is acceptable and reduces anxiety to allow a clear thought process for critical thinking.

Having a Plan

Personal observations have noted how many small emergency departments have no specific plans for intubation. Establishing a checklist and assigning duties before the incident occurs will lead to success.

Knowing Your Airway Basics

The basics of airway management are taught in most books and medical programs, but I have found that many clinicians lose this skill over time. A good practitioner will know the basics of ventilation and importance of using proper equipment to maintain successful procedures.

- Before intubation, you need the following:
  - A proper ventilation device and knowledge to use it properly
  - Proper preoxygenation before intubation
  - A review of the equipment checklist to verify equipment is available and working
  - Adequate staff knowledgeable of assigned duties

Bag-Valve Mask (BVM) Ventilation: Good Laryngoscopy, but Bad Ventilation Skills

This chapter emphasizes details about the use of a bag-valve device, because it is considered a difficult piece of equipment to properly use. The use of a bag-valve device is certainly acceptable, but placing the patient on a ventilator should be the ultimate goal.

- Dr. Rebuen Strayer discusses how ventilation is the most important skill in airway management and a provider with excellent intubation skills but average ventilation skills results in bad outcomes. Providers must remember that if you are able to ventilate a patient, then even after a failed intubation attempt, there is time to decide the next plan of action. When you are unable to ventilate a patient, then you have entered what is considered the airway death spiral.

Bag-Valve Mask Education

The use of a bag-valve mask comes from the world of anesthesiology and is the most common tool found for ventilation. The common CE technique taught to hold a BVM is not the best in emergent situations or when used by clinicians outside the operating room. Remember, anesthesiologists are generally the only people handling the airway in a controlled environment and perform the procedure almost daily. Patients having surgery generally have a preop performed and have fasted. Emergency rooms are presented with patients who are at risk for aspiration and require the clinician to perform a rapid assessment and procedure that is not frequent in rural areas.

Thumbs-Down BVM Technique

- Use both thumbs and palms to manipulate mask.

- Use both sets of forefingers to bring the mandible anterior to the maxilla (jaw thrust).

The thumbs-down technique is superior over other methods because this allows both hands to be on the mask, which is the skill part of the procedure. This allows feeling for recognition of air leaks and manipulation of the mask and jaw to correct. This also uses the strong muscles of the hands to reduce fatigue.

Additional Accessories

- The use of oral and nasal airways is declining. These devices allow for optimal air flow and minimize gastric insufflation with the risk of aspiration. Using appropriately sized oral and nasal airways each time you ventilate a patient will improve oxygenation and ventilation.

If the provider is still finding ventilation difficult, then consider inserting an airway-rescue device such as the laryngeal mask airway (LMA). LMAs are generally simple to place and directly cover the glottis opening and can be more effective than holding a mask seal.

Important Accessories for a Bag-Valve Device

- Pressure gauge / manometer—provides visual ventilation pressure
- PEEP Valve—simple device to increase alveolar recruitment and oxygenation
- EtCo2—represents ventilation to assist rate and volume

Considerations of Positive Pressure from Mechanical Ventilation

Positive Pressure

- Drives fluid out of the lungs
- Decreases preload
- Decreases cardiac output
- Decreases blood pressure

What Are the Causes of High Intrathoracic Pressure?

- Positive pressure from manual BVM or ventilator
- Chest injury

Positive Pressure from the Bag-Valve Mask

Positive pressure is caused each time you squeeze the bag and can increase when ventilation rates increase. BVM-delivered air can vary between brands and technique. The general range of BVMs is 800–2,000 ml. When considering tidal volumes at 6 ml/kg, a patient weighing 70 kg would require initial tidal volume settings at 420 ml. Most manufactured BVMs provide a minimum of 800 ml of tidal volume when the device is fully compressed, which would require the clinician to pay close attention to bag compression to prevent high intrathoracic pressure.

Prevention of High Intrathoracic Pressure When Using a Bag-Valve Mask

- Pay attention to lung compliance.

- Observe chest rise and fall.
- Use a manometer.
- Rule out chest injury such as a hemothorax or pneumothorax.

Common Intubation Mistakes

The skill of intubation is not a hard technique when the fundamentals of the procedure are learned. Like anything we do, whether it's golfing or exercising, we must learn the basic fundamentals if we expect to see a positive end result. I personally learned that going to a golf course for the first time and swinging a golf club as hard as possible didn't send the golf ball flying where I wanted. After a few lessons of golf-swing basics, I was able to hit the ball better and continuously improve. Many times, I have witnessed a clinical student being allowed to intubate a patient without any former training on the procedure and wonder how he or she expects the procedure to go well. I recently walked in a hospital to transport a patient who was being intubated after a motor-vehicle accident. My first observation had me witnessing a student attempting to advance a laryngoscope in the mouth of a patient who had a cervical collar tightly in place. I knew he would either give up or cause trauma to the patient's airway and felt I needed to intervene and help set up the student for success. I was able to stop the student and explain the need to loosen the cervical collar while I help manual cervical alignment to allow the mouth and jaw to open to advance the laryngoscope. The disheartening part of the scenario was the fact that there were two emergency-room physicians, several nurses, and a respiratory therapist present and not one person attempted to intervene.

Reason Why Many Clinicians Have Unsuccessful Intubations

- Rushed/frantic laryngoscopy
- Laryngoscopy without a plan
- Don't just stick the blade in and hope to see cords
- Poor tongue control
- No tongue on right side of blade
- Poor ergonomics
- Poor handle control, body position

Anatomic and Physiologic Considerations between Adults and Pediatrics for Intubation

Pediatric patients requiring intubation cause increased stress for many clinicians, which can result in delays for interventions and increase the opportunity for errors. Having medication and equipment size references are a must for any clinician to improve the intubation success. The below points outline anatomical differences and considerations when considering intubation for a pediatric patient.

- Adult trachea is 12–15 cm versus newborn at 4 cm, requiring special attention to ETT depth.
- Pediatric glottic opening is more anterior.
- Pediatric tongue compared to oral cavity is larger.
- Pediatric epiglottis is larger and less developed, making an indirect lift in the vallecula with a curved blade difficult.

- Children have a small functional residual capacity (FRC) and higher oxygen consumption, which can cause a rapid oxygen desaturation
- Current guidelines recommend cuffed endotracheal tubes in which the provider initially cannot inflate the cuff but has the option to inflate the cuff if there is a noted leak.

Endotracheal Tube-Size Considerations

- Reference guide to consider
    - Tube-size estimations
        - Fit through nose or compare pinky finger
        - Age in years, and then add 16 and divide by 4
        - Oral tube length
            - Age in years divided by 2 + 12 cm
            - Nasal intubations: add 3 cm to total length
            - Tube size multiplied by 3 can give a general tube depth

Making the Decision to Intubate

The decision to intubate can depend on several variables. Patient presentation has long been a quick way to know the condition of your patient. When working EMS, paramedics and EMTs assess the scene quickly and know the call may not be as serious when they see the patient on the front porch with his suitcase in hand versus face-down in the front yard. In almost any circumstance, the patient's presentation, ability to maintain a patient airway, and clinician's assessment of the airway play a vital role when deciding if the patient needs intubation.

- Rapidly assess the need and urgency for airway intervention.
- Determine the best algorithm for management.
- Pharmacology—determine which medications, what order, and what dose.
- Plan—have a backup plan.

Pediatric Reference						
KG	**Tube**	**Laryngoscope Blade**	**Oral Gastric Tube**	**Chest Tube**	**Fluid Bolus**	**Maintenance Fluid per HR**
1	3.0	0	5–8	10–12	20	4.1
2	3.0	0	5–8	10–12	40	8.3
3	3.0	0	5–8	10–12	60	12.5
4	3.0	0	5–8	10–12	80	16.5
KG	**Tube**	**Laryngoscope Blade**	**Oral Gastric Tube**	**Chest Tube**	**Fluid Bolus**	**Maintenance Fluid per HR**
5	3.0	0	5–8	10–12	100	21
6	3.5	1	8–10	12–14	120	25
7	3.5	1	8–10	12–14	140	29
8	3.5	1	8–10	12–14	160	33
9	3.5	1	8–10	12–14	180	38
10	3.5	2	8–10	14–16	200	42
11	3.5	2	8–10	14–16	220	46
12	3.5	2	8–10	14–16	240	50
13	4.0	2	10	16–20	260	54
14	4.0	2	10	16–20	280	58
15	4.0	2	10	20–24	300	63

16	4.0	2	10	20–24	320	67
17	4.5	2	12	20–24	340	71
18	4.5	2	12	20–24	360	75
19	4.5	2	12	24–32	380	79
20	5.0	2	12	24–32	400	83
21	5.0	2	12	24–32	420	88
22	5.0	2	12	24–32	440	92
23	5.0	3	14	24–32	460	96
24	5.0	3	14	24–32	480	100
25	5.0	3	14	24–32	500	104
26	5.0	3	14	24–32	520	108
27	5.0	3	14	24–32	540	113
28	5.0	3	14	24–32	560	117
29	5.5	3	14	28–32	580	120
30	5.5	3	14	28–32	600	125

Important Tips for the Clinician Who Occasionally Intubates

- Positioning the patient to provide the best view of the airway is the most important.
- Checklists are vital to eliminate forgetting equipment, medications, and dosages.
- Discuss an airway plan with your team well before a patient arrives requiring intubation.
- Consider delaying for help when faced with a potential difficult airway.
- Waveform capnography is a standard of care and instrumental in endotracheal tube confirmation and optimal ventilation.

Preoxygenation

Any patient who may require endotracheal intubation should be given high-flow oxygen immediately. Giving oxygen in anticipation of intubation has several important effects. In addition to improving the patient's oxyhemoglobin saturation, high-flow oxygen displaces nitrogen in the patient's lungs. "Washing out" the nitrogen and replacing it with oxygen convert the lung's functional residual capacity into an oxygen reservoir. Preoxygenation also increases oxygen stores in the blood and tissues. The combined effect is to enable patients to tolerate a longer period of apnea without oxygen desaturation.

The important concept is that preoxygenation provides a longer period before clinically significant desaturation, regardless of the patient's condition. The duration of this period varies greatly, depending upon patient attributes, and continuous monitoring of oxyhemoglobin saturation by pulse oximetry is essential. When assessing oxygen saturation, remember that pulse oximetry readings obtained with a finger probe may lag behind the central arterial circulation, particularly in critically ill patients

Researchers have characterized the expected time to desaturation after apnea is induced in properly preoxygenated patients of various ages and comorbid conditions. A healthy 70 kg adult can maintain oxygen saturation above 90 percent for approximately eight minutes. Young children typically fall below the 90 percent threshold in less than four minutes. The oxygen saturation of adults with severe illness or obesity and pregnant women nearing the end of their third trimester falls below 90 percent in less than three minutes despite optimal preoxygenation

Time to desaturation in emergency practice is often more rapid than anticipated. Strategies to maximize preoxygenation are as follows.

Proper positioning: For patients not immobilized for possible spinal injury, oxygenation is improved by placing them in a twenty-degree head-up position. Alternatively, thirty-degree reverse Trendelenburg positioning (bed kept straight but angled with patient's head up) may be used for immobilized patients.

Passive oxygenation during apnea: During the apneic period of RSI, provide oxygen via nasal cannula at a flow rate of 5 L/minute or at 10 L/minute. According to several randomized trials, this technique extends the period of adequate oxygen saturation during apnea, reduces the incidence of hypoxemia, and may improve outcomes

Adjuncts for airway patency: If necessary, patency of the upper airway can be maintained with adjuncts (nasal or oropharyngeal airways) and positioning maneuvers (chin lift and/or jaw thrust). The chin lift is not used when spinal precautions are being observed.

Preoxygenation with positive pressure: For patients who are unable to achieve oxygen saturation above 93 percent despite high-flow oxygen and who are judged able to tolerate positive pressure support, preoxygenation delivered via a positive-pressure device (e.g., CPAP) may enhance apnea time. Disposable positive end-expiratory pressure (PEEP) valves that can be attached to a standard bag-valve mask are available, in addition to standard positive-pressure devices.

- Administer the highest possible concentration of oxygen via the best available means.
- Remember that the traditional nonrebreather (NRB) mask provides about 70 percent oxygen when attached to a standard wall spigot set at a flow rate of 15 L/minute.
- A properly configured bag-valve-mask unit can provide 90 to 100 percent oxygen during active breathing, even without bag assist.

Alternatively, eight vital capacity breaths may be used in cooperative patients and will provide equivalent preoxygenation in less than one minute.

Bibliography

Joffe, A. M., S. Hetzel, and E. C. Liew. "A Two-Handed Jaw-Thrust Technique Is Superior to the One-Handed 'CE-Clamp' Technique for Mask Ventilation in the Apneic Unconscious Person." *Anesthesiology* 113, no. 4 (2010): 873–79.

Weingart, Scott. "Emcrit.org." Podcast 65 audio, January 22, 2012. https://emcrit.org/podcasts/bvm-ventilation.

3

Airway Algorithms and assessment

Using checklists and algorithms can provide a systematic approach to better prepare clinicians to handle a variety of airway scenarios. "Rapid-sequence intubation" (RSI) is a common term used when intubating patients, but the exact definition is misunderstood. In my experience, many clinicians administer the same sedative and paralytic agent for every intubation without consideration of the patient's condition and adverse effects that may result. Clinicians must consider all aspects of the patient's comorbidities, current medical conditions, and potential harm when taking the patient's ability to breathe. Understanding and preparing for common airway algorithms can improve success and prevent unwarranted hypoxia or death.

Overview Algorithm

The overview algorithm is a general guideline to systematically decide how to handle airways. An important note is that all paths lead to the failed airway algorithm.

Common Airway Algorithms

- Rapid-sequence intubation
- Drug-assisted intubation
- Difficult physiologic airway
- Difficult airway
- Awake airway
- Crash airway
- Failed airway

Rapid-Sequence Intubation

Rapid-sequence intubation is defined as administration after oxygenation of a potent induction agent followed by a neuromuscular blocking agent (NMBA) to induce unconsciousness and paralysis. This commonly known algorithm is misinterpreted as the standard way of intubation, although there is no standardization between facilities, and medications and techniques are provider dependent.

- The clinician must assume patient hasn't fasted and there is a high risk for aspiration.
- Rapid-sequence intubation is the technique of choice when difficult airway ruled out.

Drug-Assisted Intubation

Drug-assisted intubation is a form of intubation without the use of a paralyzing agent. States vary regarding prehospital EMS allowance of paralyzing agents, and the hospital providers should determine the local EMS protocols. For example, Mississippi protocols only allow paramedics licensed as critical-care paramedics through a Mississippi-approved program to administer paralyzing agents, and other states, such as Tennessee, allow paramedics to administer paralyzing agents after an eighty-hour course. Paramedics who are licensed as critical-care paramedics and work for a licensed critical-care transport program have the opportunity for a robust set of protocols to include chest thoracotomy, surgical airways, and arterial line placement.

Local EMS Considerations When Transferring Patients by Ground

- Determine the local EMS's capabilities (medications/ventilator capabilities).
- Sending a nurse or respiratory therapist will be helpful.
- Prepare the patient by initiating sedation and pain infusions and not just administering a paralyzing agent for convenience.

Difficult Physiologic Airway

This airway algorithm focuses on the physiological aspects of managing the patient before and during intubation. Patients with increased opportunity for cardiac arrest have certain predictors such as altered hemodynamics, oxygenation, and pH. This algorithm will assist with improving patient conditions before, during, and after intubation to minimize adverse events.

Physiologic Killers: HOp

- **H**ypotension—it is already present or can be caused by the intubation
- **O**xygenation—patient is already hypoxic or minimal oxygen reserve available

- **pH**—patient in severe metabolic acidosis or potential ICP issues from a neurological insult

Physiologic Killers (Hypotension)

Strategies to avoid cardiac arrest as a result of hypotension require strategic care to improve hemodynamics before intubation. The bullet points below provide important points a clinician must consider when faced with a hypotensive patient needing intubation.

- Intravascular access with large bore IVs or intraosseous must be available.
- Fluid resuscitation needs to be attempted to provide adequate perfusion volume.
- Aim for a higher-than-normal blood pressure (SBP ≥140 mmHg).
- Administer lower-dose sedatives and higher-dose NMBAs.
- Have push-dose pressures prepared before initiating the intubation.

Reduce Sedation Dose

Sedation is an important part of the process, but it can work against you in the hemodynamically unstable patient. Careful attention to reducing the sedative dose is important to reduce the side effects of hypotension.

Sedative of Choice (Ketamine)

- Simultaneous sympathetic surge and pain control can prevent hypotension (caution in catecholamine-depleted patients such as cold-stage sepsis).

- Dissociative dose is 1–2 mg/kg IV.
- For shock patients, reduce dose to 0.25-0.5 mg/kg IV.

Increase Paralytics

- It will take more time for NMBAs to work due to low perfusion, and increasing the NMBA dose will improve onset to paralysis.
- Adding positive-pressure ventilation to the mix will increase intrathoracic pressure causing a reduction in venous return, which will result in a reduction in cardiac output. A ventilator is preferred with special attention to airway pressures.

Paralytic of Choice (Rocuronium)
Dosed at 1.6 mg/kg IV will give the same onset of muscle relaxation as succinylcholine and longer safe apnea time.

At the Social Media and Critical Care (SMACC) Conference in 2013, Cliff Reid called this combination of low-dose ketamine and higher-dose rocuronium "rocketamine."

Push-Dose Pressors
Use of epinephrine as a push dose will prevent intubation delays and provide a quick option to improve perfusion.

- Possesses alpha and beta properties
- Increases blood pressure and cardiac output

Mixing and Dosing of Push-Dose Epinephrine.

- Take a 10 cc syringe of NS, and get rid of 1 cc (9 cc left in syringe).

- Draw up 1 cc of code-dose epinephrine (100 mcg/mL).
- This gives you 10 mcg/mL of epinephrine.
- Dosing: 0.5–2 mL (5–20 mcg) q 2–5 minutes

Options: Improving Hemodynamics

- Don't forget the basics (i.e., IVF).

Intervention 1

- Use rocketamine, dose-induction agents.
- Use sedatives low and paralytic agents high.

Intervention 2a

- Use push-dose epinephrine (alpha and beta).
- Consider push-dose phenylephrine (pure alpha).

Intervention 2b

- Consider infusion vasopressors prior to intubation.
  - Phenylephrine
  - Levophed

Intervention 3
If time permits, perform an awake intubation using a tongue depressor and EZ-Atomizer.

- Maintains endogenous catecholamines that may be suppressed by induction agents

- Increases cardiac output and maintains vascular tone
- Improves venous return

Physiologic Killers (Hypoxemia)

Hypoxia is a common reason for the need to intubate and provide supplemental oxygenation. The mechanism of acute hypoxemic respiratory failure is commonly due to disturbances in alveolar-capillary gas exchange, such as pneumonia, acute respiratory distress syndrome (ARDS), and cardiogenic or noncardiogenic pulmonary edema. Clinicians must attempt to preoxygenate when time allows to saturate hemoglobin with oxygen and maximize partial pressure of arterial oxygen before intubation.

Think "NO DESAT" (nasal oxygen during efforts securing a tube).

- Use a nasal cannula and nonrebreather at 15 LPM.
- Continue using the nasal cannula during the intubation.

If you cannot get the O_2 saturation ≥95 percent, then consider the following:

- Lung shunt physiology (i.e., pulmonary edema, pneumonia, etc.): These patients still need oxygen but will also need PEEP to recruit atelectatic alveoli to overcome the shunt.

Intervention 1: NC 15 LPM + BVM 15 LPM + PEEP Valve 5–15 cm H_2O

- No need to bag these patients, but they do need a tight seal and jaw thrust (i.e., apneic continuous positive airway-pressure [CPAP] recruitment).

Bottom line: In critically ill patients in which you cannot get O_2 saturation ≥95 percent, consider shunt physiology, and use apneic CPAP recruitment.

Intervention 2: Delayed-Sequence Intubation (DSI)

- Procedural sedation for the procedure of preoxygenation
- Give 1 mg/kg IV ketamine > preoxygenate > paralyze the patient > apneic oxygenation > intubate

Physiologic Killers (Ph)

Patients being intubated with severe metabolic acidosis can lose their respiratory compensation if not appropriately ventilated. The provider must pay close attention to minimize the acidotic state, when time allows, to minimize cardiac arrest.

Should Sodium Bicarbonate Be Administered?

Sodium bicarbonate takes hydrogen and metabolizes to CO_2, and generally patients are already hypercarbic, requiring them to blow off more CO_2 when receiving bicarb. The administration of bicarb may move the acidosis from intravascular to intracellular. This may help on a temporary basis, but it will not correct the overall problem.

Intervention 1

Attaching a ventilator and using a noninvasive positive-pressure mode help provide ventilatory support to the patient to assist blowing off CO_2 and reduce patient fatigue. EtCo2 monitoring is a must to evaluate ventilatory improvement during the preintubation period.

- NIPPV mask and actual ventilator (not BiPAP unit)
- Trained staff to use the ventilator
- SIMV mode
- TV 550 or 6 mg/kg of ideal body weight
- FiO_2 100 percent
- Flow rate 60 LPM (determines how quickly breath is delivered)
- Positive end-expiratory pressure (PEEP) 5
- Pressure support 5–10
- Set respiratory rate to 0, or set a minimum back up rate.
- Continue NIPPV mode during the RSI period.
- Once intubation meds have been administered, change respiratory rate to 12, and perform jaw thrust to help open the airway during the apneic period.
- Maintain jaw thrust until the patient is completely paralyzed.
- Once ETT placement is confirmed, change respiratory rate to 30 and Tv to 6 ml/kg of ideal body weight.

Difficult-Airway Algorithm

The difficult-airway algorithm is designed to provide identifying predictors to determine the increased potential of difficult airways. This algorithm has four dimensions that use mnemonics to help the provider remember. If you are unable to intubate or oxygenate, time is limited, and you must make a quick decision, ask these questions:

- Can I place a supraglottic airway?
- Do I have time to perform a surgical airway?

Four Dimensions

- Difficult laryngoscopy
- Difficult bag-valve-mask
- Difficult secondary airway
- Difficult cricothyrotomy

Difficult-Airway Predictors

- Immobilized trauma patient
- Combative patient
- Children and infants
- Short neck
- Prominent upper incisors
- Receding mandible
- Limited jaw opening, limited cervical mobility
- Upper-airway conditions
- Facial, laryngeal trauma

The LEMON mnemonic is a commonly used difficult-airway predictor. Many fields of medicine to include anesthesia, emergency rooms, and critical-care transport providers use this mnemonic as a routine predictor to quickly assess for difficulty managing an airway.

- Look externally
- Evaluate 3-3-2
- Mallampati score
- Obstruction
- Neck mobility

Look Externally (L)
Characteristics

- Obese
- Short neck
- Long neck
- Infants

The case below gives an example of a common and serious scenario that happens in prehospital and hospital settings and the use of proper difficult-airway predictors to assist in improving airway-management success. Angiotensin-converting enzyme (ACE) inhibitors are the leading cause of drug-induced angioedema in the United States because they are so widely prescribed and account for 20 to 40 percent of emergency-room visits. The clinician must be prepared to act quickly to prevent a total-airway occlusion and a forced invasive-airway procedure that might have been prevent.

Case Study

4:00 a.m.: Fifty-five-year-old female presents to small rural emergency department with chief complaint of tongue swelling that started at 3:00 a.m. Noted altered slurred speech secondary to abnormal tongue but able to verbalize primary complaint.

Medical history: Hypertension, diabetes, anxiety, bronchitis
Drug allergies: Cipro

Primary assessment: Alert and oriented, no respiratory distress, lungs clear, no peripheral edema
Initial vitals: BP 183/94, HR 103, SpO_2 99 percent on room air, RR 20, temp. 37C°
Home medications: Xanax, metformin, Lisinopril, albuterol
What would be your initial concerns?

Initial treatment:

- ACE-inhibitor-induced angioedema (ACEI-AAG) accounts for about a third of angioedema cases presenting to the emergency department.
- There should be a high index of suspicion for ACEI-AAG for any patient with angioedema who is taking an ACE inhibitor.
- This is often treated incorrectly, with a medication regimen directed against allergic angioedema (i.e., corticosteroids and antihistamines).
- There is a higher incidence among women and a fivefold-higher incidence among African Americans.

Clinical Features That May Help Differentiate ACEI-AAG from Histamine-Mediated Allergic Angioedema:

- Lack of allergic trigger (in contrast, ACEI-AAG may occur after minor trauma)
- Starts with focal swelling (e.g., isolated swelling of tongue or lips, often asymmetric)

- Evolves over hours (slower progression than histamine-mediated angioedema)
- Absence of urticaria or itching
- Failure to respond to antihistamines, steroid, and epinephrine
- The current treatment regimen using steroids, antihistamines, and epinephrine are ineffective for ACEI-AAG. International consensus on hereditary and acquired angioedema.
- ACEI-AAG is due to impaired metabolism of bradykinin.

Treatment:

(Currently there may not be any universal "standard therapy" for ACEI-AAG).

- Fresh frozen plasma (FFP)
    - o FFP contains multiple enzymes that degrade bradykinin, addressing the underlying disorder in ACEI-AAG.
    - o FFP has similarly been found to be effective in other forms of bradykinin-mediated angioedema such as C1-esterase deficiency.
    - o Consider early administration of 2–4 units FFP.
    - o There is no level-I evidence studies demonstrating the effectiveness of FFP.
- Catibant (FIRAZYR)
    - o Small peptide that blocks bradykinin receptors
    - o Extremely expensive ($23,000 for 30 mg, but costs may vary)

Another form of angioedema can be hereditary in nature and requires a different approach. In many cases, the patient or family members have been properly educated and prescribed the appropriate medication, but clinicians must understand the urgency and be able to quickly have another plan in place.

An Overview of Hereditary Angioedema Diagnosis:

- Hereditary-angioedema patients (HAE) usually have normal results on most routine laboratory tests.
- During attacks of gastrointestinal edema, abdominal radiographs may demonstrate features of ileus in HAE patients.
- Abdominal ultrasonography or computed tomography may show edematous thickening of the intestinal wall, a fluid layer around the bowel, and large amounts of free peritoneal fluid.
- Chest radiographs may demonstrate pleural effusions.

Treatment:

- Berinert, a C1-esterase inhibitor (human), is used in adults and children to treat swelling and/or painful attacks of HAE affecting the abdomen, face, or throat.
- FFP seems to be safe and effective in preventing exacerbations of HAE before surgery and for acute exacerbations of HAE without evidence of it initiating an attack or worsening a preexisting attack.

Evaluate the 3-3-2 (E)

- Can three fingers fit between the incisors?
    - o A mouth that can open that far has good temporomandibular joint mobility.
- Mandible length can be measured by evaluating three fingers from the mentum to the hyoid bone?
    - o Less than three fingers demonstrates a potential anterior glottic opening.
    - o Either more or less than three fingers makes ventilation increasingly difficult.
- Distance from the hyoid to the thyroid tells you something about neck length—two fingers' distance is ideal.
    - o More than two fingers demonstrates a distant glottic opening which may require a miller blade for length.

Mallampati Score (M)

If the patient can cooperate, ask her to stand, open the mouth, stick out the tongue, and say, "Ah." The structures that are visible compose Mallampati class I (the easiest airway), II, III, or IV (most difficult). If you see the tonsillar pillars, that's Mallampati class I. If all you can see is the palate, that's class IV.

Obstruction (O)

- Perform an external visual assessment.
- Look for anything that might get in your way.
- The enemies of airways include soft tissue swelling from smoke inhalation, burns, broken necks, trauma to the face

or neck, foreign bodies in the airway, and excessive soft tissue from obesity.

Neck Mobility (N)

- Practice with a C-collar to understand the limited anatomical manipulation and visual availability when a C-collar is applied.
- Patient positioning has been proven to increase intubation success.
- Align three planes of view to include the trachea, pharynx, and oropharynx to achieve maximum view of important airway anatomy.

***Neck mobility is desirable. Unfortunately, many patients who need resuscitation in the emergency department arrive in neck braces or compromised neck mobility, and you may not be able to move them into preferred positions for establishing a definitive airway.

***Shoulder and head elevation by any means that brings the patient's sternum onto the horizontal plane of the external auditory meatus maintains or improves laryngoscopic view significantly.

There are many pneumonic descriptions available to help the clinician quickly rule out or identify problems that may arise. Each time you are faced with an airway situation, the mnemonic or some other proven predictors should be considered when time is feasible.

Difficult BMV: MOANS

M: Mask seal should ideally be performed by one provider while the other provider concentrates on ventilation. Wet substances or facial hair increases the difficulty of holding a mask seal.

O: Obesity/obstruction refers to chest wall and abdomen weight from obesity or pregnancy and can make ventilation more difficult increasing the risk of gastric insufflation and rapid desaturation of oxygen.

A: Age—loss of muscle and tissue tone may not allow the mask to seat firmly on the face to prevent leakage of air.

N: No teeth will make a mask seal more difficult.

S: Stiff lungs with poor pulmonary compliance will make ventilation more difficult and increase gastric insufflation.

Difficult Secondary Devices: RODS

R: Restricted mouth opening make inserting a laryngoscope (direct or indirect) difficult.

O: Obstruction/obesity make a secondary airway difficult at times due to not directly ventilating past the vocal cords in the trachea. A supraglottic device may be difficult to seal, and using an indirect ventilation device, such as a King airway, will general require higher airway pressures

D: Disrupted or distorted airway will increase airway resistance similar to a patient with obstruction or obesity. The severity of airway resistance will depend on the severity of the distorted airway.

S: Stiff necks or jaws will limit visualization and displacement of airway anatomy.

Difficult Cricothyrotomy: SMART

S: Surgery (recent/remote)

M: Mass

A: Access/anatomy

R: Radiation

T: Tumor

Airway Assessment

- Body habitus: Obesity requires precise preplanning for optimal airway view and consideration of ventilation due to adipose tissue on chest increasing opportunity for higher airway pressures.

- Blood/secretions: Always prepare for fluid or blood in the airway. Not being prepared can delay successfully intubating and potentially cause pulmonary issues later.
- C-spine: Remove the C-collar to allow opening of the airway. Always have someone available to maintain C-spine immobilization if possible.
- Intubated before (especially children): Parents can be a good resource if the child has been previously intubated and possibly advise if the airway is difficult.
- Mallampati score: Although mentioned previously, this isn't always optimal.

Bibliography

Brown, N. J., S. Byiers, D. Carr, M. Maldonado, and B. A. Warner. "Dipeptidyl Peptidase-IV Inhibitor Use Associated with Increased Risk of ACE Inhibitor-Associated Angioedema." *Hypertension* 54, no. 3 (2009): 516–23. https://doi.org/10.1161/hypertensionaha.109.134197.

Cook, T. M., N. Woodall, J. Harper, and J. Benger. "Major Complications of Airway Management in the UK: Results of the Fourth National Audit Project of the Royal College of Anaesthetists and the Difficult Airway Society. Part 2: Intensive Care and Emergency Departments†." *BJA: British Journal of Anaesthesia* 106, no. 5 (2011): 632–42. https://doi.org/10.1093/bja/aer059.

Forsythe, Sean M., and Gregory A. Schmidt. "Sodium Bicarbonate for the Treatment of Lactic Acidosis." *Chest* 117, no. 1 (2000): 260–67. https://doi.org/10.1378/chest.117.1.260.

Gangadharan, Lakshmi, C. Sreekanth, and Mabel C. Vasnaik. "Prediction of Difficult Intubations Using Conventional Indicators; Does Rapid Sequence Intubation Ease Difficult Intubations? A Prospective Randomised Study in a Tertiary Care Teaching Hospital." *Journal of Emergencies, Trauma, and Shock* 4, no. 1 (2011): 42. https://doi.org/10.4103/0974-2700.76836.

Heffner, Alan C., Douglas S. Swords, Marcy N. Neale, and Alan E. Jones. "Incidence and Factors Associated with Cardiac Arrest Complicating Emergency Airway Management." *Resuscitation* 84, no. 11 (2013): 1500–4. https://doi.org/10.1016/j.resuscitation.2013.07.022.

Heffner, A. C., D. S. Swords, M. L. Nussbaum, J. A. Kline, and A. E. Jones. "372 Predictors of the Complication of Post-Intubation Hypotension during Emergency Airway Management." *Annals of Emergency Medicine* 60, no. 4 (2012): S132. https://doi.org/10.1016/j.annemergmed.2012.06.404.

"The HOP Mnemonic for Difficult Airway Physiology." EMCrit. Last modified June 3, 2017. https://emcrit.org/emcrit/hop-mnemonic/.

Hung, Orlando R., and Michael F. Murphy. Management of the Difficult and Failed Airway Review Questions. New York: McGraw-Hill Medical, 2012.

Jackson, C. "High Tracheotomy and Other Errors—The Chief Causes of Chronic Laryngeal Stenosis." *The American Journal of the Medical Sciences* 162, no. 3 (1921): 444. https://doi.org/10.1097/00000441-192109000-00028.

Kheterpal, S., L. Martin, A. M. Shanks, and K. K. Tremper. "Prediction and Outcomes of Impossible Mask Ventilation." *Survey of Anesthesiology* 53, no. 6 (2009): 266. https://doi.org/10.1097/sa.0b013e3181be863b.

Mississippi State Department of Health. "Regulations & Protocols—Mississippi State Department of Health." Mississippi State Department of Health—Home. Accessed November 20, 2016. http://msdh.ms.gov/msdhsite/_static/47,0,305.html.

Mosier, Jarrod, Raj Joshi, Cameron Hypes, Garrett Pacheco, Terence Valenzuela, and John Sakles. "The Physiologically Difficult Airway." *Western Journal of Emergency Medicine* 16, no. 7 (2015): 1109–17. https://doi.org/10.5811/westjem.2015.8.27467.

Reed, M. J. "Can an Airway Assessment Score Predict Difficulty at Intubation in the Emergency Department?" *Emergency Medicine Journal* 22, no. 2 (2005): 99–102. https://doi.org/10.1136/emj.2003.008771.

Riedl, Marc. "Hereditary Angioedema Therapies in the United States: Movement toward an International Treatment Consensus." *Clinical Therapeutics* 34, no. 3 (2012): 623–30. https://doi.org/10.1016/j.clinthera.2012.02.003.

Roberts, James R., and Richard C. Wuerz. "Clinical Characteristics of Angiotens in Converting Enzyme Inhibitor-induced Angioedema." *Annals of Emergency Medicine* 20, no. 5 (1991): 555–58. https://doi.org/10.1016/s0196-0644(05)81616-6.

Stewart, M., and R. McGlone. "Fresh Frozen Plasma in the Treatment of ACE Inhibitor-induced Angioedema." *BMJ Case Reports 2012* 2012 (2012): pii: bcr2012006849-bcr2012006849. https://doi.org/10.1136/bcr-2012-006849.

Walls, Ron, and Michael Murphy. *Manual of Emergency Airway Management.* Philadelphia, PA: Wolters Kluwer Health, 2012.

Weingart, Scott. "Podcast 3—Laryngoscope as a Murder Weapon (LAMW) Series—Ventilatory Kills—Intubating the Patient with Severe Metabolic Acidosis." EMCrit. Last modified May 2, 2016. https://emcrit.org/emcrit/tube-severe-acidosis/.

Weingart, Scott D., and Richard M. Levitan. "Preoxygenation and Prevention of Desaturation During Emergency Airway Management." *Annals of Emergency Medicine* 59, no. 3 (2012): 165–75.e1. https://doi.org/10.1016/j.annemergmed.2011.10.002.

4

Equipment Overview

MEDICAL-DEVICE MANUFACTURERS OFFER new airway products at reasonable prices that provide innovative ways to successfully manage airways. No specific device will always guarantee success, and providers should have more than one device available. Ideally, having a device that will surround the glottis (laryngeal mask airway) and intubate the esophagus for indirect ventilation (King/Combitube) would offer alternative ways to ventilate patients if direct laryngoscopy is unsuccessful. This section will review commonly seen airway devices with no specific endorsement of any device. Keep in mind that this covers a small portion of the devices available.

Know how to use the devices that are stocked at your facility.

Adjuncts/Alternative Devices

- Combitube/EOA
- Laryngeal mask airway
- King

- Salt
- Airtraq
- Cric/trach
- Video laryngoscope (indirect laryngoscopy)

Esophageal Intubating Devices (Indirect Ventilation)

The Combitube and King airways are supraglottic airways that are inserted blindly and consist of a curved tube with ventilation apertures located between two inflatable cuffs. The Combitube requires cuff inflation from separate valves with a dual lumen tube in the event a tracheal intubation occurs. The King airway offers a single valve/pilot balloon to inflate both cuffs with a tracheal intubation unlikely. The distal cuff seals the esophagus; the proximal cuff seals the oral pharynx. Both airways have the same contraindications for patients who have a gag reflex, known esophageal disease (e.g., cancer, varices, stricture), laryngectomy with a stoma, and/or caustic ingestion or airway burns.

Combitube

This airway device offers a blind insertion opportunity with twin lumens to allow ventilation in the trachea or esophagus, although tracheal intubation with this device occurs in less than 5 percent of patients.

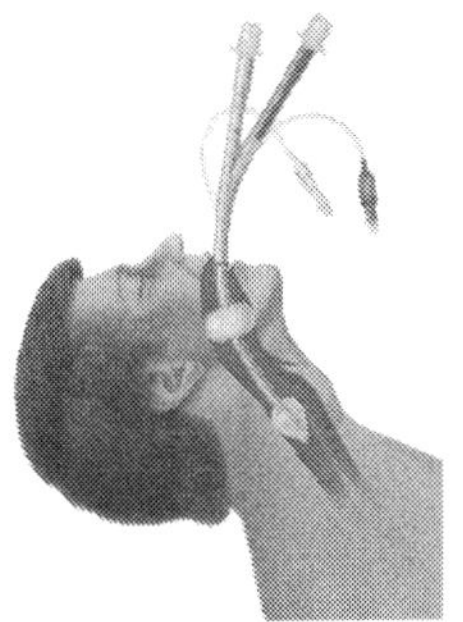

- Blinded insertion
- Two lumens to inflate
- Two cuffs (distal and proximal)
- Esophagus: intended use
- Trachea: <5 percent insertion
- Limited sizes
    - o 37F (small) 4′ to 5′6″ height
    - o 41F (tall) >5′6″
- No pediatric sizes

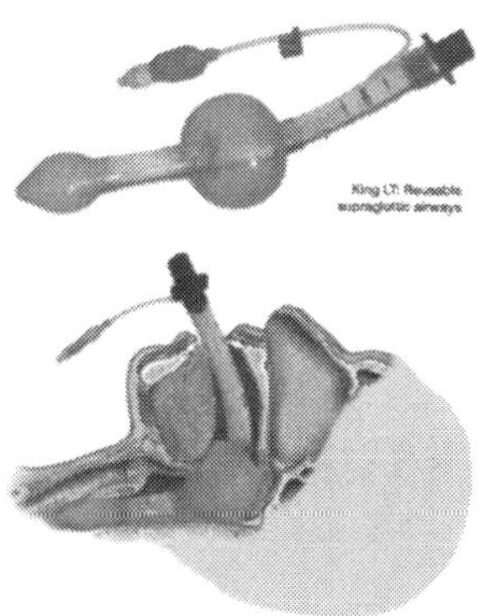

King Airway (Laryngeal Tube Airway)

- Curved design decreases the chance of the tube going into the trachea.
- Blind insertion
- Single lumen
- Inflates both balloons simultaneously
- Potential to lose cuff pressure
- Quick insertion
- Size available for pediatric and adults

Laryngeal Mask Airway (LMA)

The LMA is a common airway used in anesthesia for its ease of use and quick placement. Newer developed supraglottic airways allow for gastric occlusion to prevent aspiration, access for endotracheal tube placement by blind insertion, and self-inflation to prevent prolonged pressure to carotids and tissues.

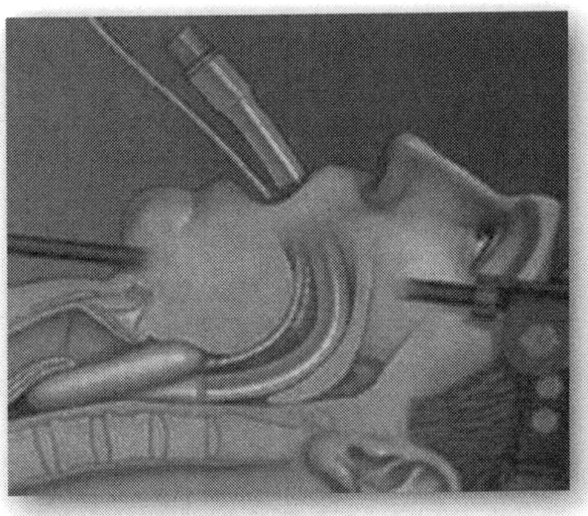

- Blind insertion.
- LMA resides in the hypopharynx, with the anterior portion of the LMA abutting the posterior aspect of the tongue.
- The epiglottis rests within the bowl of the mask in an anatomical position in most situations.
- This mask provides no protection from aspiration.

Intubating Supraglottic Airway

- Sizes from adult to infant.
- Allows the passage of a standard endotracheal tube through the air-Q. This allows the air-Q to be placed initially and

then it can act as a conduit for intubation, without removing the air-Q.

- Small ramp in outlet directs the endotracheal tube toward the glottic opening.

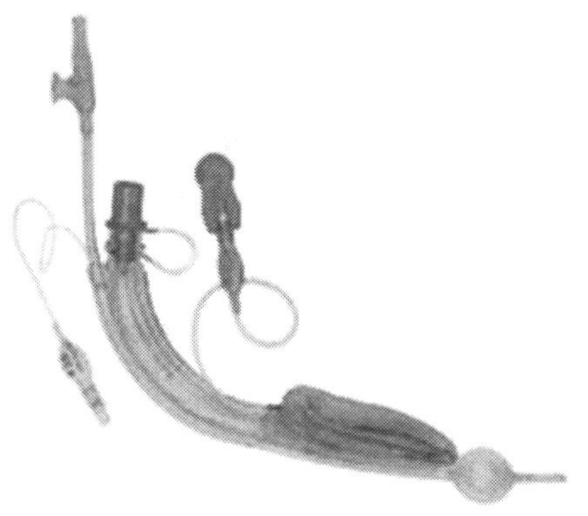

Video Laryngoscope

The use of video laryngoscopes has become a popular choice with intubation. Many have differences of opinion on which device should become the first line item used. Rather than calling them video laryngoscopes, think of the process as direct versus indirect intubation. The video laryngoscopes have multiple blade options, but the Macintosh blade is the most common, giving an anterior view versus a standard blade with direct view. Both direct or indirect options require training to become comfortable with and understand how each one differs.

> The most common problem identified in many hospitals is the lack of training on how to manipulate the endotracheal tube when using a video laryngoscope with a good anterior view.

Video Laryngoscope Facts

- Eliminates direct line of sight
- Provides acute anterior view
- Magnifies airway anatomy
- Uses a different technique compared to direct laryngoscopy
- Allows for recording
- Should not be first line unless difficult airway expected

***Remember "cheers versus beers" when considering technique differences between direct and indirect laryngoscopy.

Cheers: Lifting handle upward and outward as if you were toasting a glass to celebrate

Beers: Lifting handle upward with a slight tilt back as if you were drinking a beer (careful to avoid damage to the teeth)

Emergency Cricothyrotomy

Cricothyrotomy is a procedure routinely discussed among clinicians, but rarely do you hear of one being performed in rural facilities or prehospital. The controversial past of this procedure was first described by Dr. Chevalier Jackson, a laryngologist at the Jefferson Medical School in Philadelphia, who often performed this procedure for severe infection or an inflammatory process (e.g., diphtheria) before antibiotics were available. This procedure was eventually condemned by Dr. Jackson after reviewing cases of tracheal stenosis. In the 1970s, two physicians reported low complication rates secondary to cricothyrotomy for prolonged mechanical ventilation and created a new enthusiasm that the procedure of cricothyrotomy was, in fact, a safe and reasonable option. Cricothyrotomy is rarely performed and requires continuous training to maintain competency. A large study performed in the United Kingdom gives examples of preventative deaths to include cricothyrotomy complications. Below is an excerpt of the study that explains important considerations regarding airway management.

Important Study Involving Airways

National Audit Project (NAP4) Study

In 2011, the Health Services Research Centre (HSRC) of the National Institute of Academic Anesthesia (NIAA) was launched, with the aim of being a hub for world-class anesthesia research (including perioperative, pain-related, and subspecialty research). Now, the responsibility for management of the NAPs has been transferred to the HSRC, with oversight by Council of the College. NAPs 1–4 were supported and managed by the Professional

Standards Department of the Royal College of Anesthetists. This study provided research to support airway management and capnography.

Website: http://www.nationalauditprojects.org.uk/

A Review of the National Audit Project (NAP4) Study

- Captured detailed reports of major complications of airway management in the United Kingdom
- Largest study of major complications of airway management ever performed
- Captured cases from all NHS hospitals in England, Scotland, Wales, and Northern Ireland
- Included cases from anesthesia, intensive-care units, and emergency departments

NAP4 Executive Summary for ICU and the Emergency Department

- One in four major airway events
- Failure to use capnography in ventilated patients likely contributed to more than 70 percent of ICU related deaths
- Displaced tracheal tubes were the greatest cause of major morbidity and mortality in ICU.
- Most events in the emergency department were complications of rapid-sequence induction.

NAP4 Executive Summary: Interpretation of Results

"Many of the events and deaths reported to NAP4 were likely to have been avoidable."

Surgical Airway Procedure

- This skill involves creating an opening in the trachea by invasive surgical means to oxygenate and ventilate.
- This is an important skill for failed airway and generally a last-resort procedure.
- When the clinician is unable to oxygenate or ventilate, this procedure must be performed precisely and rapidly.
- There are conflicting studies debating which technique is fast and safe.

Surgical Technique Options

- Seldinger technique
- Scalpel
- Scalpel, bougie guided

***There are many available surgical airway kits on the market. Identify which one is available in your department. State regulations vary regarding EMS scope of practice.

Commercial Surgical Airway Kits

- Rusch QuickTrach
- Pulmodyne Control-Cric

- Portex Cricothyrotomy Kit
- Melker Cuffed Emergency Cricothyrotomy Catheter Set (Seldinger)

Identifying Landmarks

Traditional Methods

- Palpation of the thyroid prominence (Adam's apple) and the gap between the lower thyroid cartilage and the cricoid ring
- Works well in thin males but not when there is significant neck tissue and musculature
- In women, the thyroid lamina is smaller and has a shallower angle; there is no thyroid prominence.

"Laryngeal handshake," by Dr. Richard Levitan

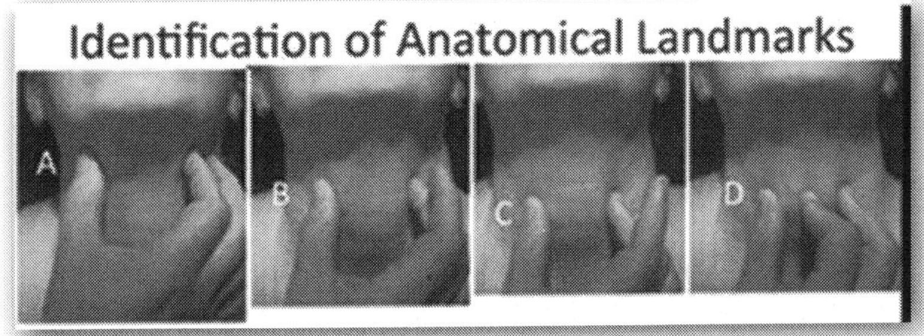

- Instead of using the tip of the index finger to feel for landmarks, palpate the laryngeal framework using the whole hand.
- The hyoid, thyroid, and cricoid form a rhomboid structure and move as a unit from side to side.
- Instead of feeling for the thyroid prominence, palpate the broad thyroid lamina.

- Palpating the firm lamina of the thyroid and moving the whole laryngeal framework from side to side will consistently confirm the landmarks.

Technique

- Start gently up high with the hyoid, using the thumb and index finger, under the angle of the mandible.
- Staying lateral to midline, slide down to the broad, firm thyroid lamina. At this point, use the index finger to come to midline and palpate the thyroid prominence in men. Lower down is the inferior cornu of the thyroid, bilaterally overlapping the cricoid cartilage. This is the bottom of the rhomboid, below which are the softer tracheal rings.
- Using the firm lamina of the thyroid as a guide (and especially if the thyroid prominence is not felt), the index finger is brought midline to the cricothyroid membrane at the inferior aspect of the lamina. In men, the thyroid cartilage is always more prominent than the cricoid, but in women they often have equal prominence.

Discussion

- What is the difference between a tracheal versus an esophageal intubation device?
- What device is not recommended in small children?
- Which failed-airway procedure appears to have better success?
- Do all laryngeal mask airways allow an endotracheal tube to be passed through?

- Which laryngoscopy maneuver generally provides a better anterior view but increased the difficulty advancing the endotracheal tube?

References

"Air-q® Airways Disposable." Mercury Medical. Accessed January 12, 2017. http://www.mercurymed.com/product-category/air-q-airways-disposable/.

Cook, T. M., N. Woodall, J. Harper, and J. Benger. "Major Complications of Airway Management in the UK: Results of the Fourth National Audit Project of the Royal College of Anaesthetists and the Difficult Airway Society. Part 2: Intensive Care and Emergency Departments." *British Journal of Anaesthesia* 106, no. 5 (2011): 632–42.

Levitan, R. Vimeo, April 15, 2015. Cricothyrotomy with laryngeal handshake, sternal stabilization Accessed January 18, 2017. https://vimeo.com/124180047.

Tumpach, E. A., M. Lutes, D. Ford, and E. B. Lerner, "The King LT versus the Combitube: Flight Crew Performance and Preference." *Prehospital Emergency Care* 13, no. 3 (2009): 324–28.

5

Low-Cost Options

Low-Cost Options

- Silk tape
- Suction catheter
- Bougie
- Two-person
- Intubate bubbles
- Double tube
- Fish hook
- Withdraw ETT stylet

***The identified options are potential ways to improve intubation success when working in an environment that has minimum airway supplies. The "redneck tricks" use commonly found items to improve success, although there is no supporting evidence available to support many items mentioned in this chapter.

Low-Budget Ideas
Silk Tape

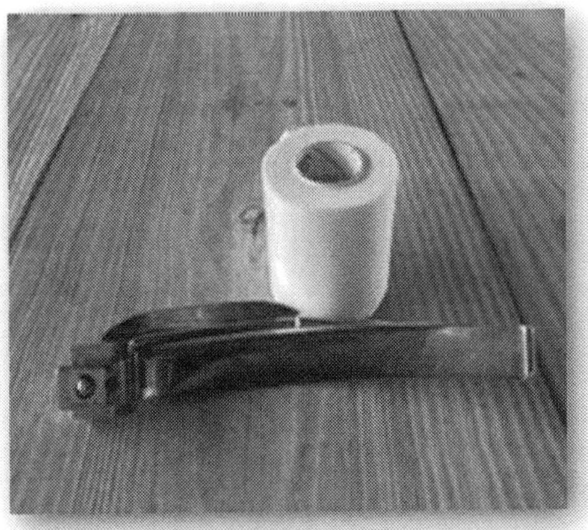

Aligning the laryngoscope blade with silk tape will help when presented with a bloody airway. This reduces slippage and allows more control.

Two-Person

There will be times when having someone gently assist lifting the laryngoscope will prevent you from losing the site of the vocal cords. Be sure they lift in a way that doesn't allow the teeth to be involved.

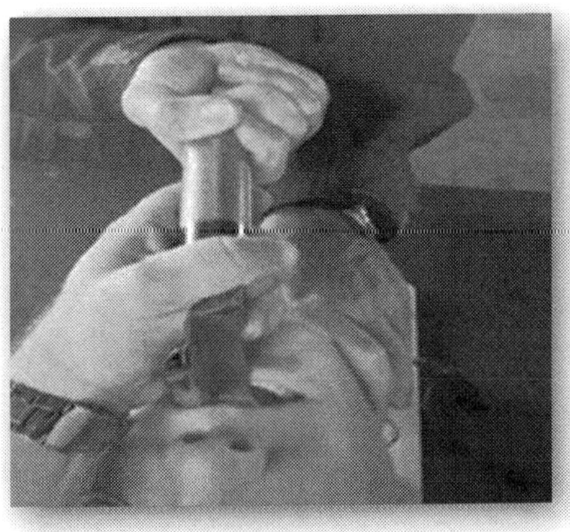

Suction Catheter

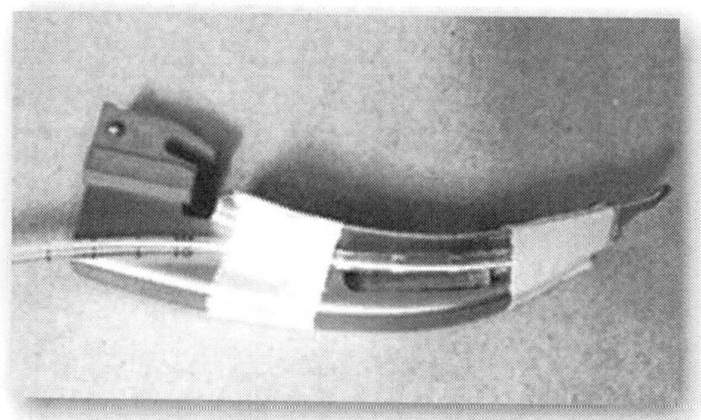

Secure a suction catheter under the laryngoscope blade to allow suctioning while displacing anatomy.

Fish Hook

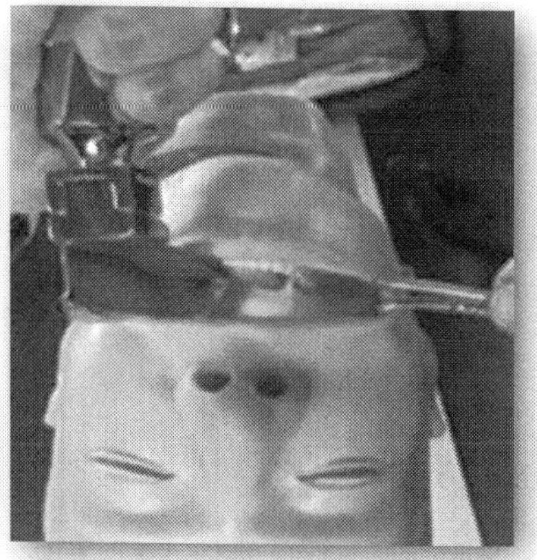

Using the appropriate-size stylet, fold the stylet in half, and gently bend near the end. This allows you to enlarge the viewing area.

Bougie

- Using a bougie is ideally a two-person procedure.
- Place bougie just anterior and midline to the arytenoids and feel for tracheal rings.
- If unable to visualize confirmation, feel for the tracheal rings.
- For a secondary confirmation, advance bougie to approximately 40 cm, and resistance should be felt as the bougie hits the carina, and/or the bougie will turn as it advances one bronchi.
- To avoid the ETT catching on the arytenoids, do not remove the laryngoscope until it is at the correct depth.
    - o If resistance is met when advancing the ETT, pull back the ETT 2 cm, and rotate counterclockwise.
        - This orients the bevel of the ETT posteriorly, and it should advance.
        - To avoid advancing the bougie to far, do not advance past the black line (if available) or 23 cm.
- Counterclockwise rotation of the ETT as it approaches the larynx will decrease chance of the ETT catching on laryngeal soft tissues.

Laryngeal vestibule: Space between the laryngeal inlet and vocal cords. This is where a bougie can hang up. Gentle twisting of bougie can allow it to safely pass.

Intubate Bubbles

- During attempts at glottis visualization, bubbles may be visualized, providing guidance for advancing a bougie or ETT.

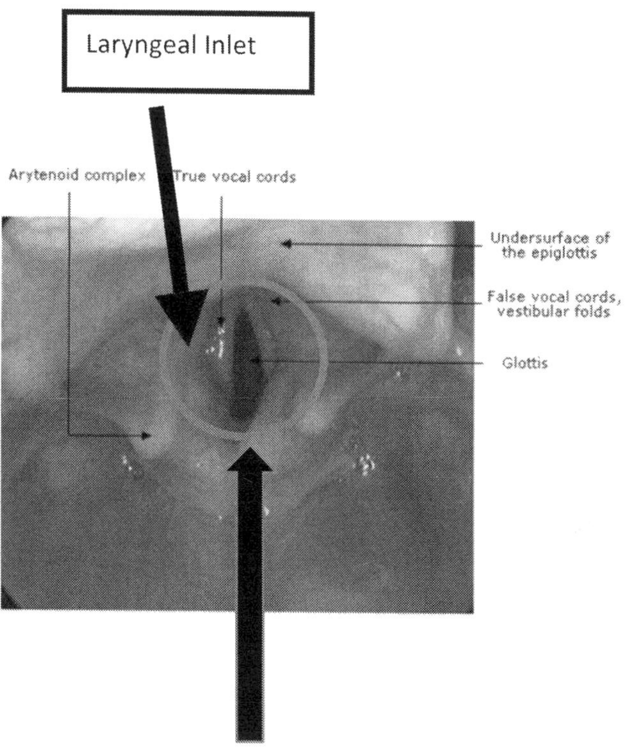

Double Tube

- If esophageal intubation is determined, the wrongfully placed ETT could be left in place and a second ETT used. The esophageal-placed ETT can prevent the provider from placing the second ETT in the same place. The clinician should use caution with this method due to the prolonged apnea that may be involved resulting in hypoxia. This should only be considered if a second ETT is already prepared and proper preoxygenation is performed.

Withdraw ETT Stylet

- With the proper-sized stylet in place, having an assistant gently withdraw the stylet from the ETT will cause the distal end of the ETT to rise anteriorly. This may be beneficial when using a video laryngoscope with an anterior airway.

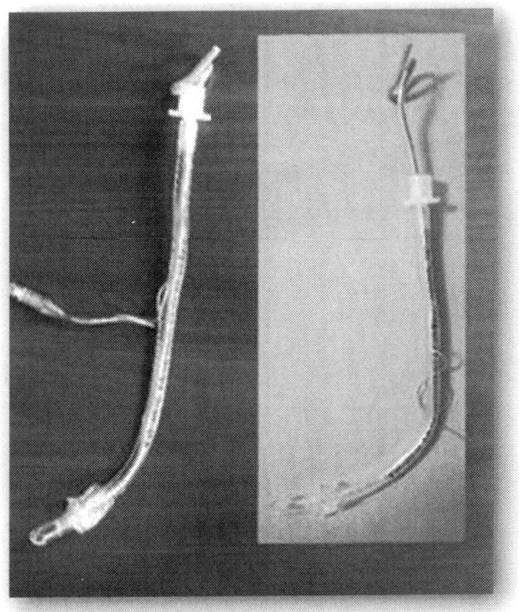

6

Pharmacology

DRUG CHOICES—WHERE DO we start? Decisions on which drug to use, when, what dosage, and when to repeat can be a difficult task if clinicians aren't prepared. Some clinicians are limited by their license and organizational policies, but many seem to lack the understanding of the importance in drug choice. Plenty of literature is available through studies for recommendations regarding pharmacology and airway management, but no hardcore policy exists within most small rural emergency departments.

It's not hard to find a paramedic or nurse who has witnessed a patient receiving a paralyzing NMBA without any pain or sedation considerations. I have personally witnessed a paralyzed but not sedated head bleed that resulted in herniation from increased intracranial pressure and a postintubation cardiac arrest from a catecholamine-induced hypoxia. Occasionally, patients receive NMBAs right before departure on a transfer to make it easier on the paramedic, or the sending physician starts an infusion that the paramedic is not familiar with. These common stories are routinely seen within rural areas, resulting in poor patient outcomes.

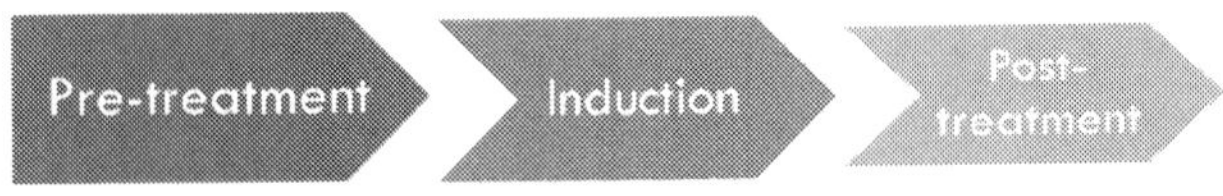

Module 1: Pretreatment

Pretreatment pharmacological agents are important to blunt the reflex sympathetic response to laryngoscopy (RSRL). Although some pretreatment agents are little data, clinicians must consider the importance of each agent in any airway scenario. Below are commonly used pretreatment agents for consideration and must be administered at least three minutes before the procedure. The clinician must consider the value versus delay of waiting to intubate the critically ill patient and some situations require immediate intubation.

Lidocaine—Amide Local Anesthetic

Little studies exist demonstrating Lidocaine's effectiveness to blunt the rise of ICP during laryngoscopy, but many clinicians continue to use it. Studies do demonstrate Lidocaine's effectiveness to reduce bronchospasms if there is little time to administer a beta-2 agonist, such as albuterol.

- Class III antiarrhythmic
- Contraindications: Allergy or high-grade heart failure or heart block

- Caution: Hepatic dysfunction or pseudocholinesterase deficiency
- Dose: 1.5 mg/kg
- Onset: 45–90 seconds

Fentanyl (Sublimaze)—Opioid Receptor Agonist

Fentanyl is an opioid receptor agonist that blunts the sympathetic response during laryngoscopy. Given as a last pretreatment drug over 30-60 seconds, Fentanyl can blunt the rise in ICP and reduce side effects of laryngoscopy for patients with heart disease. Hemodynamically compromised patients may be dependent on sympathetic responses, so careful consideration must be taken to reduce hypotension during intubation.

- Onset: 60–90 seconds
- Adult dose: 2–3 mcg/kg
- Pediatric dose: 2–3 mcg/kg
- Duration: 30–60 minutes
- Side effects: Respiratory depression
- Muscle-wall rigidity
    - Related to dose and speed of administration
    - Generally more common in high doses
    - Reversal using naloxone or short-acting neuromuscular blocking agent

Atropine—Anticholinergic Agent; Antidote; Antispasmodic Agent

Atropine use as a pretreatment before intubation is documented as an off-label use but commonly used in the emergency and transport setting. Keep in mind that pediatric patients develop bradycardia early as a result of hypoxia, and atropine will mask any bradycardia, resulting in clinicians delaying ventilations.

- Blocks vagal stimulation during laryngoscopy
- Excessive salivation inhibitor
- Acceptable for use in children one year
- RSI pretreatment dose: IV: 0.01 to 0.02 mg/kg (minimum of 0.1 mg)
- Inhibit salivation: IM, IV, SubQ: 0.4 to 0.6 mg

Module 2: Induction Agents

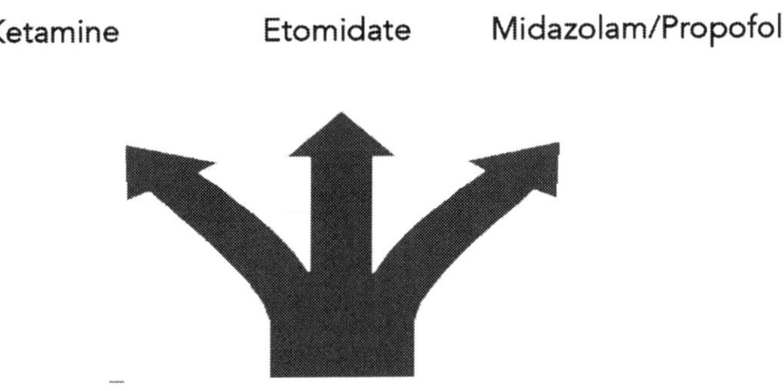

Induction or sedative agents are an integral part of the intubation process to include drug selection and dosage based on patient presentation and stability. Clinicians using the same pharmacological choice no matter what type of patient presentation are increasing the odds for sentinel events. My good friend L. J. Relle once told an audience that not being prepared gets you a "one-way ticket on the fail-boat." Although I laugh at his statement, poor pharmacological choices are personally witnessed often, and my personal experience demonstrates that clinicians are desensitized to poor outcomes.

When considering induction agents, one must ask several questions related to the patient condition to help decide the desired outcome. What's the best drug to use? Ultimately, the desired drug of choice should have a rapid onset, cause unconsciousness, and result in amnesia with minimal hemodynamic effects. There are many drugs available that fit some of these criteria, but there is no specific drug that is a "one does all." Each time a clinician is faced with intubating a patient, each drug should be carefully considered of the benefits versus risks. Why do we sedate and what are some common drugs used for induction? Below are commonly used induction agents to consider, but understand there are many more drugs used in different settings and geographical locations.

Etomidate (Amidate)—Hypnotic

Etomidate is an imidazole-derived agent that was first reported and published in 1965. Initially developed as an antifungal agent, the potent hypnotic activity of several compounds was noted during animal testing and appeared safer than barbiturates. Adrenal toxicity was noted in the 1980s, which diminished published studies of etomidate, but the use in the emergency intubation setting has increased over the past several years. Etomidate should be considered a push-dose drug and not recommended as an infusion.

- Adult dose: 0.3mg/kg
- Pediatric dose: Not recommended
- Onset: 14–45 seconds

- Duration: 3–12 minutes
- Do not give multiple doses or infusion.

Etomidate Pros:

- Rapid onset
- Hemodynamically stable
- It does not inhibit sympathetic tone or myocardial function, which results in minimal changes in blood pressure or heart rate. This is especially important with patients with heart disease or hemorrhagic shock.
- It has cerebroprotective properties by limiting cerebral blood flow and lowering cerebral oxygen demand making it safe for patients with elevated ICP.

Etomidate Cons:

- Not FDA approved for children
- Adrenal suppression has been a major controversy and careful consideration must be used with sepsis type patients.
- No blunting of the sympathetic-stress response to upper-airway stimulation from a laryngoscope. Consider lidocaine and opioids prior to etomidate administration.

Ketamine (Ketalar)—Phencyclidine Derivative

Ketamine is a dissociative anesthetic agent similar in structure to phencyclidine (PCP). Ketamine provides minimal effect on the respiratory drive and contains analgesia, amnestic, and sedative effects. Ketamine is considered a superior induction agent due to the rapid onset accompanied by analgesia and sedation. Patients with reactive airway disease benefit from ketamine's bronchodilation from catecholamine release. There are still controversial arguments about ketamine's effects on elevated ICP, but the evidence is weak.

- Adult dose: 1–2 mg/kg
- Pediatric dose: 1–2 mg/kg
- Onset: 45–60 seconds
- Duration: 10–20 minutes

Ketamine Pros:

- Rapid onset
- Most hemodynamically stable induction agent
- Causes catecholamine release making it attractive for hypotensive patients
- Preservation of upper-airway reflexes making it a good choice for difficult airway or awake intubation

Ketamine Cons:

- Reemergence phenomenon exists when patients experience disturbing dreams when awaking from ketamine-induced anesthesia. Many clinicians use a form of benzodiazepine to help minimize this occurrence.
- Potential adverse effects from catecholamine-depleted patients

Propofol (Diprivan)—Hypnotic

Propofol is a short-acting intravenous sedative-hypnotic that was first available for commercial use in the United States in 1989. This medication has been an induction agent of choice for the anesthesia world in the operating room and a favorite for conscious sedation. Although propofol is commonly used by anesthesia for intubation, the emergency setting limits the benefits of the use of propofol due to the hemodynamic side effects. The manufacturer recommends avoiding rapid push doses for the elderly or hemodynamically unstable patient to avoid vasodilation and myocardial depression.

1,000 mg in 100 ml Propofol 10 mcg/kg/min	
Weight	**Pump rate**
5 kg	0.3
10 kg	0.6
15 kg	0.9
20 kg	1.2
25 kg	1.5
30 kg	1.8
35 kg	2.1
40 kg	2.4
45 kg	2.7
50 kg	3
55 kg	3.3
60 kg	3.6
65 kg	3.9
70 kg	4.2
75 kg	4.5
80 kg	4.8
85 kg	5.1
90 kg	5.4
90 kg	5.7

- Dose: Adults: Rapid bolus: 1.5 mg/kg
  - o Elderly and unstable: Not recommended
  - o Initial infusion: 5–20 mcg/kg/min
  - o Titrate dose quickly up to 50 mcg/kg/min
- Onset: 15–45 seconds
- Duration: 5–10 minutes

Propofol Pros:

- Excellent for stable patients
- Agent of choice for pregnant patients
- Short acting
- Rapid onset

Propofol Cons:

- Strong vasodilation/hypotension
- Myocardial depression
- Decrease in cerebral perfusion

Benzodiazepines

- Midazolam (Versed)
- Lorazepam (Ativan)
- Diazepam (Valium)
- Not a good choice for RSI due to slow onset of action
- Still commonly used, but there are better induction drugs available

Midazolam (Versed)

- The most commonly used benzodiazepine used for induction
- Not a good induction choice but can be useful for seizure patients
- Dose: 0.2 mg/kg—expect moderate drop in blood pressure
- 0.25 to 1 mcg/kg/minute
- Onset: 60–90 seconds
- Duration: 15–30 minutes

Neuromuscular Blocking Agents (NMBAs)

Neuromuscular blocking agents (NMBAs) block the binding of acetylcholine (ACh) to the motor endplate. They are divided into depolarizing or nondepolarizing agents based upon their mechanism of action. The primary purpose of using NMBAs is to prevent aspiration, and clinicians must remember that they provide no sedation or analgesia. The use of NMBAs without proper sedation and analgesia can produce harmful effects in certain situations, and careful attention must be placed on evaluating if the patient is properly sedated. The most commonly used NMBAs will be discussed.

Succinylcholine (Anectine, Quelicin)

Succinylcholine is a depolarizing (noncompetitive) neuromuscular blocking agent that is a favorite NMBA of choice due to its rapid onset and short duration of paralysis. Clinicians must remember that it is better to overestimate doses to assure full paralysis. Patients who are only partially paralyzed will be more difficult to intubate and potentially have adverse hemodynamic effects.

- Contraindications: Family history of malignant hyperthermia (MH) or neuromuscular disorders (muscular dystrophy)
- Adverse effects: Hyperkalemia
- Adult dose: 1.5 mg/kg
- Pediatric dose: 1 mk/kg
- Onset: 45 seconds
- Duration: 6–10 minutes

Nondepolarizing Agents

Categorized Groups

- Benzylisoquinoline and aminosteroid compounds

Aminosteroid Compounds

- Vecuronium
- Pancuronium
- Rocuronium
- Aminosteriod (most common due to no histamine release)

Rocuronium (Zemuron)

Rocuronium was introduced in the United States in 1994 and designed to be a weaker antagonist at the neuromuscular junction than pancuronium. Rocuronium is a derivative of vecuronium and doesn't require reconstitution.

- Blocks the action of ACH
- Best competitive agent
- Adult dose: 1 mg/kg
- Pediatric dose: 0.9 to 1.2 mg/kg
- Onset: 60 seconds
- Duration: 40–60 minutes

Vecuronium (Norcuron)

- Requires reconstitution
- Adult Dose: 0.1 mg/kg
- Pediatric Dose: 0.08 to 0.1 mg/kg
- Onset: 75–90 seconds
- Duration: 60–75

Pancuronium (Pavulon)

- Not a good choice for RSI
- Slow onset
- Causes tachycardia

<u>Remember the Following Sequence</u>

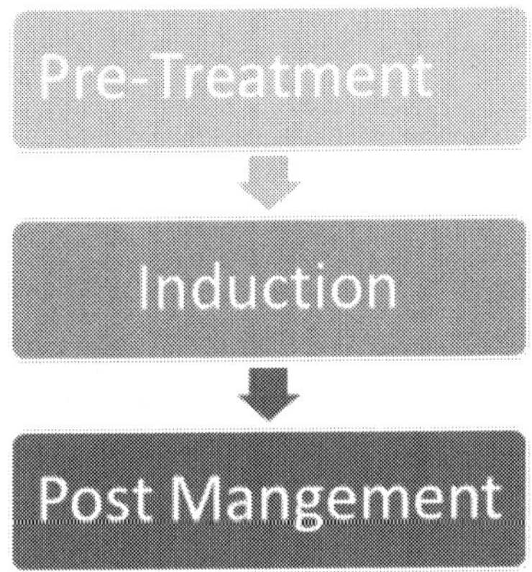

7

Postintubation Management

ONCE A CLINICIAN has performed a successful intubation, it is imperative that a prevention of an unplanned extubation checklist is performed. It would be terrible to successfully intubate a normal or difficult airway only to be called in emergently to reintubate or manage a cardiac arrest for a displaced endotracheal tube. Proper sedation and pain management postintubation is also just as important as the initial intubation. Poorly sedated and pain-managed patients not only experience a nightmare-type scenario, but they can also result in poor hemodynamic outcomes.

- Continue pain and sedation management optimize pain first and then sedation. Can you imagine feeling terrible pain but unable to move or wake up? This happens and causes a sympathetic response that can have adverse effects. Expect a patient without proper pain and sedation management to have an increasing blood pressure, heart rate, and tearing.

- Consider using a pain scale such as the Richmond Agitation-Sedation Scale (RASS). This can be an easy way to allow the staff taking care of the patient to adjust.
- Only paralyze when needed and not for convenience.
- Consider infusions for continuous pain and sedation management, and use push boluses for quick results.
- Secure the endotracheal tube well. Be careful to not cause harm when using a commercial device.
- Place a nasogastric or oral gastric tube.
- Elevate the head of bed to reduce ventilator acquired infections and improve lung mechanics.
- Place commercial head blocks or rolled towels on either side of head to reduce movement.
- Place in-line suction if available.
- Verify EtCo2 is being used.
- Verify endotracheal tube depth and recheck often.
- Perform postintubation blood gases, and adjust ventilator settings accordingly.
- Keep a bag-valve mask at bedside, and verify the mask is attached.

Postintubation Management Infusions

- Fentanyl infusion dose: 25–150 mcg/hour
- Propofol infusion dose: 5–50 mcg/kg/min
- Ketamine infusion dose: 0.05–0.4 mg/kg/hour
- Midazolam infusion dose: 0.25–1 mcg/kg/minute

ABOUT THE AUTHOR

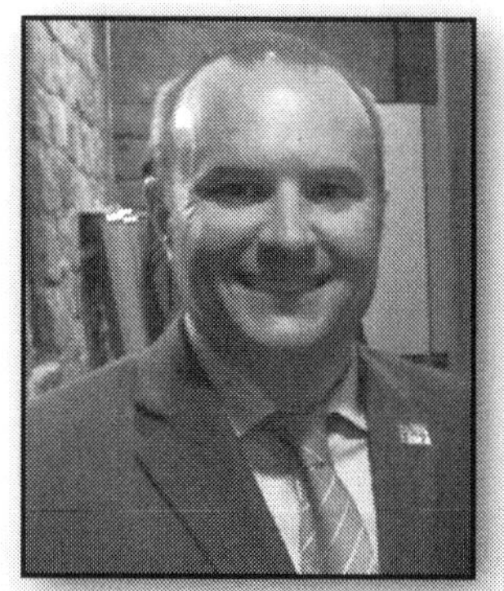

Sam Marshall is a flight paramedic and operations manager of two remote helicopter bases for the University of Mississippi Medical Center. Sam brings over twenty years of EMS and critical-care experience; he started his career working as an EMT basic at a local EMS service. Sam completed paramedic school while employed as an EMT/firefighter and graduated critical-care paramedic school a few years later.

Sam holds advanced certifications to include Critical-Care Paramedic (MS-CCP), Certified Neonatal and Pediatric Transport (C-NPT), and Certified Flight Paramedic (FP-C) with his most recent accomplishment including graduation from the Medical Transport Leaders Institute's medical-transport executive course (CMTE).

After an airway-related death of a close friend, Sam focused on improving airway management through research and education, including partnering with the EC-Healthnet Family Residency Program, which added this course to its curriculum.

Sam was born and raised in Mississippi and continues to live in his hometown with his wife of seventeen years, Danielle, and two daughters, Maggie and Cate.

Made in the USA
Lexington, KY
09 January 2018